LUNG CANCER DIET PLAN COOK BOOK

A Handbook of the Lung Cancer Diet: Good Cooking for Lung Cancer Patients

REX LEWIS

Table of Contents

Introduction

Lung Cancer Is A Form Of Cancer That Originates In The Cells Of The Lungs, Essential Organs That Oxygenate The Blood. There Are Two Primary V Categories of Lung Cancer: Non-Small Cell Lung Cancer (NSCLC) And Small Cell Lung Cancer (SCLC). Non-Small Cell Lung Cancer (NSCLC) Is A Prevalent Kind Of Lung Cancer That Encompasses Various Subtypes, Including Adenocarcinoma, Squamous Cell Carcinoma, And Large Cell Carcinoma. Small Cell Lung Cancer (SCLC) Is Less Prevalent But Has A Tendency To Proliferate And Metastasize Quickly.

The Main Cause Of Lung Cancer Is Tobacco Smoke, Which Includes Exposure To Secondhand Smoke. Additional Risk Factors Comprise Exposure To Environmental Toxins Including Radon Gas And Asbestos, A Familial History Of Lung Cancer, And Specific Genetic Variables. Although Lung Cancer Can Impact Both Smokers And Non-Smokers, The Risk Is Notably Elevated In Smokers.

Nutrition Is Essential For The Prevention, Treatment, And Overall Health Of Persons With Lung Cancer. A Nutritious Diet Can Complement Medical Treatment And Assist In Managing The Negative Effects Of Cancer Medicines, While It Cannot

Replace Them. Here Are Some Essential Aspects Concerning Nutrition And Lung Cancer:

• Maintaining An Optimal Weight Is Crucial As It Might Affect The Prognosis And Treatment Results For Individuals With Lung Cancer. It Is Crucial To Maintain A Balanced Diet To Achieve A Healthy Weight.

• Adequate Protein Consumption Is Essential For Persons With Lung Cancer, Particularly Those Receiving Cancer Treatment. Protein Aids In Preserving Muscle Mass, Bolstering Immunological Function, And Promoting Tissue Repair.

• Foods High In Antioxidants, Such Fruits And Vegetables, Can Assist In Fighting Oxidative Stress And Inflammation. Vitamins Such As A, C, And E Contribute To Bolstering The Immune System.

• Hydration Is Critical For Overall Health, Especially During Cancer Treatment To Prevent Worsening Side Effects Such As Fatigue And Nausea.

• Omega-3 Fatty Acids Found In Fatty Fish, Flaxseeds, And Walnuts Can Have Anti-Inflammatory Properties And Promote General Well-Being.

• Reduce Consumption Of Processed Foods, Sugary Snacks, And Excessive

Red Or Processed Meats. Emphasizing Entire, Nutrient-Rich Diets Is Favored.

• Personalized Approach: Nutritional Requirements Can Differ Depending On An Individual's Cancer Type, Treatment Regimen, And General Health. Seeking Advice From A Qualified Dietitian Or Nutritionist Helps Customize Dietary Suggestions To Meet Individual Needs.

Individuals With Lung Cancer Should Collaborate With Their Healthcare Team, Including Oncologists And Nutrition Professionals, To Create A Customized And Balanced Diet Plan That Supports Their Overall Cancer Treatment.

CHAPTER ONE
Basics of a Lung Cancer Diet

A Lung Cancer Diet Aims To Supply Vital Nutrients To Promote General Well-Being, Sustain Energy Levels, And Address Possible Adverse Effects Of Cancer Therapies. Individual Dietary Requirements Can Differ, Thus It Is Advisable To Consult With Healthcare Specialists, Especially A Licensed Dietitian Or Nutritionist. Here Are Some Fundamental Aspects Of A Diet For Lung Cancer:

• **Balanced Diet:** Aim for a Balanced Diet That Includes A Variety Of Nutrient-Dense Foods From All Food Groups. This Includes Fruits, Vegetables, Whole Grains, Lean

Proteins, And Dairy Or Dairy Alternatives.

• **Protein Intake:** Adequate Protein Is Essential For Maintaining Muscle Mass, Supporting Immune Function, And Aiding In Tissue Repair. Good Sources Of Protein Include Lean Meats, Poultry, Fish, Eggs, Dairy Products, Legumes, Nuts, And Seeds.

• **Fruits and Vegetables:** Incorporate A Variety Of Colorful Fruits And Vegetables Into The Diet. These Foods Are Rich In Vitamins, Minerals, And Antioxidants, Which Can Help Support The Immune System And Fight Oxidative Stress.

• **Whole Grains:** Choose Whole Grains Such As Brown Rice, Quinoa, Whole Wheat, Oats, And Barley. These Provide Fiber, Vitamins, And Minerals That Contribute To Overall Health.

• **Healthy Fats:** Include Sources Of Healthy Fats, Such As Avocados, Nuts, Seeds, And Olive Oil. Omega-3 Fatty Acids, Found In Fatty Fish Like Salmon And Flaxseeds, May Have Anti-Inflammatory Benefits.

• **Hydration:** Stay Well-Hydrated By Drinking Plenty Of Fluids, Such As Water, Herbal Teas, And Clear Broths. Proper Hydration Is Important For Managing Side Effects Like Fatigue And Nausea.

- **Small, Frequent Meals:** Eating Smaller, More Frequent Meals Throughout The Day May Be Easier To Tolerate, Especially For Individuals Experiencing Appetite Changes Or Digestive Issues Due To Cancer Treatments.

- **Limit Processed Foods:** Minimize The Intake Of Processed Foods, Sugary Snacks, And High-Fat Or Fried Foods. These Choices May Contribute To Inflammation And May Not Provide Optimal Nutritional Support.

- **Supplements:** Depending On Individual Needs, Healthcare Providers May Recommend Specific Supplements, Such As Vitamin D, Calcium, Or Nutritional Supplements,

To Address Any Deficiencies Or Support Overall Health.

- **Consultation with Healthcare Professionals:** Work Closely With Healthcare Professionals, Including A Registered Dietitian, To Tailor Dietary Recommendations To Individual Circumstances, Treatment Plans, And Side Effects.

Nutritional Requirements Can Differ, And Dietary Changes May Be Needed Depending On How Individuals Respond To Therapies And Their Overall Health Condition. Establishing Clear Communication With Healthcare Professionals And Emphasizing A Balanced And Nutritious Diet Are

Crucial Elements In Aiding Patients With Lung Cancer.

Foods to Include In a Lung Cancer Diet

Incorporating A Range Of Nutrient-Rich Food Into A Diet For Lung Cancer Can Supply Vital Nutrients, Promote General Well-Being, And Assist In Handling Possible Adverse Effects Of Cancer Therapies. Here Are Some Foods To Consider:

• **Lean Proteins:** Chicken, Turkey, Fish (Such As Salmon And Tuna), Lean Beef, Eggs, Tofu, Legumes (Beans And Lentils), And Low-Fat Dairy Products Provide Important Protein For Muscle Maintenance And Immune Support.

• **Colorful Fruits And Vegetables:** Include A Variety Of Fruits And Vegetables Rich In Vitamins, Minerals, And Antioxidants. Examples Include Berries, Citrus Fruits, Leafy Greens, Carrots, Sweet Potatoes, Broccoli, And Bell Peppers.

• **Whole Grains:** Choose Whole Grains For A Good Source Of Fiber, Vitamins, And Minerals. Examples Include Brown Rice, Quinoa, Whole Wheat Bread, Oats, And Barley.

• **Healthy Fats:** Incorporate Sources Of Healthy Fats, Such As Avocados, Nuts (Like Almonds And Walnuts), Seeds (Flaxseeds And Chia Seeds), And Olive Oil. These Fats May Have Anti-Inflammatory Benefits.

• **Fatty Fish:** Fatty Fish, Such As Salmon, Mackerel, And Sardines, Are Rich In Omega-3 Fatty Acids, Which May Have Anti-Inflammatory Properties.

• **Dairy Or Dairy Alternatives:** Choose Low-Fat Or Non-Fat Dairy Products Or Fortified Dairy Alternatives For A Source Of Calcium And Vitamin D. Examples Include Milk, Yogurt, And Fortified Plant-Based Milk Alternatives.

• **Hydrating Foods:** Include Hydrating Foods Like Water-Rich Fruits (Watermelon, Cucumber, Oranges), Clear Broths, And Herbal Teas To Help Maintain Hydration.

- **Ginger and Mint:** Ginger And Mint May Help Alleviate Nausea, A Common Side Effect Of Cancer Treatments. Consider Incorporating Ginger In Teas Or Adding Mint To Dishes.

- **High-Fiber Foods:** Foods High In Fiber, Such As Whole Grains, Fruits, Vegetables, And Legumes, Can Aid In Digestion And Help Manage Constipation, Which Can Be A Side Effect Of Certain Treatments.

- **Small, Frequent Meals:** Eating Smaller, More Frequent Meals Throughout The Day May Be Easier To Tolerate For Individuals Experiencing Changes In Appetite Or Digestive Issues.

- **Probiotic Foods:** Probiotic-Rich Foods Like Yogurt with Live Cultures, Kefir, Sauerkraut, and Kimchi May Help Support Gut Health.

• **Herbs and Spices:** Utilize Herbs And Spices To Enhance The Taste Of Dishes Without Depending On Excessive Salt. For Instance, Turmeric, Garlic, And Cinnamon Possess Potential Anti-Inflammatory Effects.

It Is Essential To Customize The Diet According To Individual Tastes, Dietary Tolerances, And Specialized Treatment Programs. It Is Crucial To Engage With Healthcare Specialists, Especially A Qualified Dietitian Or Nutritionist, To Ensure That The Diet Is Tailored To Specific Nutritional

Requirements And To Address Any Possible Issues Or Inadequacies.

CHAPTER TWO
Foods to Avoid or Limit

Individuals With Lung Cancer, Particularly Those Receiving Treatment, May Need To Avoid Or Limit Specific Foods To Manage Symptoms And Promote General Health. Individual Tolerance Levels Might Vary, Therefore Suggestions May Vary Depending On Certain Situations. It Is Essential To Get Advice From Healthcare Specialists, Such As A Qualified Dietitian, For Tailored Recommendations. Here Are Some Overarching Principles On Foods To Steer Clear Of Or Restrict:

• **Processed Foods:** Limit Your Intake Of Processed Foods, Which Are

Generally High In Salt, Sugar, And Bad Fats. These Can Increase Inflammation And May Not Give Adequate Nutritional Support.

- **High-Fat and Fried Foods:** Reduce The Consumption Of High-Fat And Fried Foods, As They May Be Harder To Digest And Can Contribute To Nausea, Especially For Individuals Undergoing Cancer Treatments.

- **Excessive Red And Processed Meats:** Limit The Consumption Of Red And Processed Meats, As These May Be Associated With An Increased Risk Of Certain Cancers. Opt For Lean Protein Sources Such As Poultry, Fish, And Plant-Based Proteins.

• **Sugary Snacks And Beverages:** Minimize The Intake Of Sugary Snacks, Candies, And Sweetened Beverages. These Foods Can Contribute To Energy Spikes And Crashes And May Not Support Overall Health.

• **Dairy Products If Lactose Intolerant:** For Individuals Who Are Lactose Intolerant Or Experiencing Digestive Issues, Limit Dairy Products. Opt For Lactose-Free Alternatives Or Discuss With A Healthcare Professional.

• **Alcohol:** Limit Or Avoid Alcohol, As It Can Interact With Medications And May Contribute To Dehydration. Alcohol Can Also Affect The Liver, And Individuals With Lung Cancer May

Already Be Dealing With Compromised Liver Function.

• Strongly Flavored Or Spicy Foods: Some Individuals May Find That Strongly Flavored Or Spicy Foods Exacerbate Nausea Or Digestive Issues. Consider Avoiding These If They Are Not Well-Tolerated.

• Large Meals: Instead Of Large Meals, Consider Eating Smaller, More Frequent Meals Throughout The Day. Large Meals May Be Harder To Digest, Especially For Those Experiencing Changes In Appetite Or Digestive Discomfort.

- **Caffeine And Stimulants:** While Moderate Caffeine Intake Is Generally Considered Safe, Individuals Experiencing Anxiety Or Sleep Disturbances May Benefit From Limiting Caffeine Intake. It's Important To Stay Well-Hydrated With Water Or Herbal Teas.

- **Raw Or Undercooked Seafood And Eggs:** To Minimize The Risk Of Foodborne Illness, Avoid Raw Or Undercooked Seafood And Eggs.

- **Certain Acidic Foods:** For Individuals With Acid Reflux Or Esophageal Irritation, Limiting Acidic Foods And Beverages, Such As Citrus Fruits, Tomatoes, And Caffeinated Drinks, May Be Beneficial.

Remember That Everyone Has Different Interests, Tolerances, And Nutritional Demands. Consultation With Healthcare Specialists, Such As A Licensed Dietitian Or Nutritionist, Is Essential For Tailoring Dietary Recommendations To The Unique Needs And Circumstances Of People With Lung Cancer.

Meal Planning and Preparation Tips

Meal Planning And Preparation Can Help Persons With Lung Cancer By Providing Nutritious, Easily Digestible Meals. Here Are Some Tips For Meal Planning And Preparation:

Consult A Dietitian:

• Seek Guidance From A Registered Dietitian Or Nutritionist Who Can Help Create A Personalized Meal Plan Based On Individual Nutritional Needs, Preferences, And Any Dietary Restrictions.

Balanced Meals:

• Plan Meals That Include A Balance Of Protein, Carbohydrates, And Healthy

Fats. This Balance Helps Provide Essential Nutrients And Energy.

Small, Frequent Meals:

• Consider Serving Smaller, More Frequent Meals Throughout The Day Instead Of Three Large Meals. This Can Be Easier To Manage For Individuals Experiencing Changes In Appetite Or Digestion.

Hydration:

• Ensure Adequate Hydration By Including Water, Herbal Teas, And Clear Broths In The Meal Plan. Staying Hydrated Is Crucial, Especially For Managing Side Effects Like Fatigue And Nausea.

Easy-To-Digest Foods:

• Choose Foods That Are Easy To Digest, Such As Cooked Vegetables, Lean Proteins, And Whole Grains. Avoid Overly Spicy Or Greasy Foods That May Cause Discomfort.

Pre-Cut And Pre-Packaged Options:

• Opt For Pre-Cut Fruits And Vegetables Or Pre-Packaged, Washed Greens To Simplify Meal Preparation, Making It More Convenient And Less Labor-Intensive.

Freeze Meals:

• Prepare And Freeze Meals In Advance. Having A Variety Of Frozen, Ready-To-Heat Options Can Be Helpful, Especially On Days When

Energy Levels Are Low Or Cooking Is Challenging.

High-Calorie And Nutrient-Dense Snacks:

• Keep Nutrient-Dense Snacks Readily Available, Such As Nuts, Seeds, Yogurt, Cheese, And Fresh Fruit. These Snacks Can Provide Additional Calories And Nutrients Between Meals.

Include Comfort Foods:

• Incorporate Comfort Foods That Are Both Nourishing And Enjoyable. This Can Help With Maintaining A Positive Relationship With Food During Challenging Times.

Collaborative Cooking:

• If Possible, Involve Family Members, Friends, Or A Caregiver In Meal Preparation. This Not Only Eases The Workload But Also Creates A Supportive Environment.

Experiment With Flavors:

• Experiment With Herbs And Spices To Enhance The Flavor Of Meals Without Relying On Excessive Salt. Some Individuals May Find That Certain Flavors Help Alleviate Nausea Or Enhance Appetite.

Keep A Food Diary:

• Keep A Food Diary To Track Preferences, Tolerances, And Any Reactions To Specific Foods. This Can

Be Helpful Information To Share With Healthcare Professionals.

Meal Delivery Services:

• Consider Using Meal Delivery Services Or Pre-Prepared Meal Options That Cater To Specific Dietary Needs. These Services Can Provide Convenient And Nutritious Options.

Flexible Planning:

• Be Flexible With Meal Plans And Adapt Them Based On Energy Levels, Appetite, And Any Treatment-Related Side Effects. Listen To The Body's Cues And Adjust As Needed.

Positive Eating Environment:

• Create A Positive And Comfortable Eating Environment. Sit Down To Enjoy Meals, Use Appealing Tableware, And Make The Dining Experience As Pleasant As Possible.

Remember That The Idea Is To Offer Nourishment While Respecting Individual Choices And Circumstances. Regular Communication With Healthcare Providers And A Qualified Dietitian Can Assist Ensure That Meal Plans Are Adapted To The Specific Needs Of Lung Cancer Patients.

CHAPTER THREE
Supplements and Nutritional Support

Supplements And Nutritional Assistance Can Be Beneficial For People With Lung Cancer, Particularly During And After Treatment. However, It Is Critical To Consult With Healthcare Specialists, Such As Oncologists And Qualified Dietitians, Before Beginning Any Supplementation Regimen. Considerations For Supplements And Nutritional Support:

• Consult Healthcare Specialists, Such As An Oncologist And Qualified Dietitian, Before Adding Supplements To The Diet. They Can Evaluate

Individual Needs And Determine Whether Supplementation Is Required.

- **Multivitamins:** Taking A Daily Multivitamin May Help Cover Nutritional Deficits. However, Unless Instructed By A Healthcare Professional, You Should Not Exceed The Recommended Daily Allowances For Vitamins And Minerals.

- **Vitamin D:** Vitamin D Promotes Bone Health And Immunological Function. Some Cancer Patients May Have Low Vitamin D Levels. Healthcare Providers Can Recommend And Supervise Supplements As Needed.

• Calcium Intake Is Crucial For Bone Health, Particularly For Those Undergoing Cancer Therapies That May Impact Bone Density. Calcium Supplements May Be Prescribed If Food Consumption Is Inadequate.

• **Omega-3 Fatty Acids:** Omega-3 Fatty Acids, Available In Fish Oil Or Algae-Based Supplements For Individuals Who Eschew Fish, May Have Anti-Inflammatory Properties. They Can Be Considered With The Assistance Of Healthcare Professionals.

• **Probiotics:** Probiotic Supplements Help Improve Gut Health, Especially For Those Experiencing Digestive Difficulties Due To Cancer Therapies.

However, Dietary Sources Of Probiotics, Such As Live Cultures In Yogurt, Should Also Be Examined.

• **Iron:** Iron Supplements May Be Prescribed For Those With Cancer-Related Anemia. However, Excessive Iron Consumption Can Be Dangerous, Thus Supplementation Should Be Managed By A Healthcare Practitioner.

• B Vitamins (B12 And Folate) Are Essential For Energy Metabolism. Cancer Treatments And Dietary Limitations May Have An Impact On B Vitamin Levels, Necessitating Supplementation.

• **Zinc:** Zinc Is Essential For Immune Function And Wound Repair. Some

Cancer Treatments May Impair Zinc Absorption, Thus Supplementation May Be Explored In Certain Circumstances.

• **Appetite Stimulants:** Healthcare Experts May Prescribe Appetite Stimulants Or Nutritional Supplements To Help Patients With Appetite Loss Maintain Proper Calorie Intake.

• **Protein Supplements:** Protein Is Crucial For Preserving Muscular Mass, Especially During Cancer Therapies. Protein Supplements May Be Recommended If Dietary Intake Is Insufficient, But It Is Critical To Select High-Quality Sources.

- **Individualized Approach:** Supplement Requirements Differ Based On Individual Health, Treatment Goals, And Dietary Habits. An Personalized Approach That Considers Various Situations Is Critical For Optimal Nutritional Support.

It's Crucial to Remember That, While Supplements Might Be Useful In Certain Cases, They're Not A Substitute For A Healthy Diet. Whole Foods Should Be The Major Source Of Nutrition Wherever Possible. Furthermore, Continued Discussion With Healthcare Providers, As Well As Regular Monitoring, Can Assist In Adjusting Supplement Regimens To

Meet The Individual's Changing Demands And Health State.

Special Considerations for Different Stages of Lung Cancer

Lung Cancer Is Typically Classified Into Various Stages According To The Severity Of The Condition. The Therapy And Nutritional Requirements For Persons With Lung Cancer May Fluctuate Depending On The Stage Of The Disease. Special Considerations For Various Stages Of Lung Cancer Are As Follows:

Early-Stage Lung Cancer (Stages I And II):

Surgery as a Primary Treatment:

• For Individuals Undergoing Surgery As The Primary Treatment, Nutritional Support Focuses On Preoperative Preparation And Postoperative Recovery. Adequate Protein Intake Is Crucial For Tissue Repair.

Emphasis on Healing Foods:

• Prioritize Nutrient-Dense Foods, Including Fruits, Vegetables, Lean Proteins, And Whole Grains, To Support Overall Health And Aid In Recovery.

Maintaining Healthy Weight:

• Focus On Maintaining A Healthy Weight To Support Optimal Recovery

And Reduce The Risk Of Complications Associated With Surgery.

Monitoring Side Effects:

• Monitor And Manage Potential Side Effects Of Surgery, Such As Changes In Appetite, Nausea, And Difficulty Swallowing, With The Guidance Of Healthcare Professionals.

• Locally Advanced Lung Cancer (Stage III):

Combination Therapies:

• Treatment Often Involves A Combination Of Surgery, Radiation Therapy, And Chemotherapy. Nutritional Support Is Essential To Manage Potential Side Effects Of These Therapies.

Addressing Radiation Side Effects:

• Individuals Undergoing Radiation Therapy May Experience Side Effects Such As Fatigue, Nausea, And Changes In Taste. Tailor The Diet To Address These Issues And Maintain Adequate Nutrition.

Protein And Calorie Needs:

• Protein And Calorie Needs May Increase During Treatment. Work With A Registered Dietitian To Ensure That Nutritional Requirements Are Met.

• Advanced Or Metastatic Lung Cancer (Stage IV):

Focus On Symptom Management:

• For Individuals With Advanced Or Metastatic Lung Cancer, The Focus May Shift Towards Managing Symptoms And Improving Quality Of Life. Nutritional Support Aims To Address Specific Concerns.

Managing Appetite Loss:

• Address Appetite Loss With Small, Frequent Meals, Nutrient-Dense Snacks, And, If Necessary, Appetite Stimulants Under The Guidance Of Healthcare Professionals.

Addressing Nausea And Digestive Issues:

• Individuals Undergoing Chemotherapy May Experience

Nausea And Digestive Issues. Choose Easily Digestible Foods And Work With Healthcare Professionals To Manage These Side Effects.

Individualized Nutritional Support:

• Tailor Nutritional Support To Individual Needs, Considering Treatment Goals, Overall Health, And Personal Preferences. This May Involve Adjusting The Diet, Incorporating Supplements, Or Exploring Alternative Feeding Methods.

End-Of-Life Care:

• In Advanced Stages, Individuals May Transition To Palliative Or End-Of-Life Care. Nutritional Goals May Shift

Towards Maintaining Comfort And Quality Of Life Rather Than Aggressive Nutritional Interventions.

Survivorship:

Recovery and Long-Term Health:

• After Completing Treatment, Individuals May Focus On Recovery And Long-Term Health. Emphasize A Well-Balanced Diet Rich In Nutrients To Support Overall Well-Being.

Monitoring For Late Effects:

• Monitor For Potential Late Effects Of Treatment, Such As Changes In Bone Health, Metabolism, Or Digestive Function. Adjust The Diet As Needed And Continue Regular Follow-Up With Healthcare Professionals.

Psychosocial Support:

• Provide Psychosocial Support To Help With Any Lasting Emotional Or Psychological Impacts From The Cancer Experience That Could Affect Appetite And Eating Patterns.

Personalized Care Is Essential At Every Phase Of Lung Cancer. Consistent Communication With Healthcare Specialists Such As Oncologists And Registered Dietitians Is Essential To Ensure That Nutritional Support Is Tailored To The Individual's Treatment Plan, Objectives, And General Health.

CHAPTER FOUR
The Importance of Exercise

Exercise Is Vital For Preserving General Health And Well-Being, And It Is Particularly Significant For Those With Lung Cancer. Integrating Consistent Physical Activity Into One's Schedule Can Bring About Numerous Beneficial Outcomes, Especially For Individuals Receiving Cancer Treatment. Here Are Some Main Arguments Emphasizing The Significance Of Exercise For Patients With Lung Cancer:

• **Enhanced Physical Function:** Regular Physical Activity Aids In Preserving And Enhancing Physical Function, Including Strength,

Flexibility, And Endurance. This Is Particularly Advantageous For Persons Who May Suffer From Muscle Weakness Or Exhaustion As A Result Of Cancer Therapies.

• **Improved Cardiovascular Health:** Participating In Aerobic Activities Like Walking, Swimming, Or Cycling Can Enhance Cardiovascular Health. It Is Crucial For General Health And Can Enhance Endurance And Stamina.

• **Weight Management:** Exercise Contributes To Weight Management By Fostering A Healthy Equilibrium Between Calorie Consumption And Expenditure. It Is Crucial To Sustain A Healthy Weight For General Well-

Being And It Could Have A Beneficial Effect On Treatment Results.

• Resistance Training Activities Aid In Developing And Preserving Muscle Strength, Which Is Crucial For Persons Facing Muscle Atrophy Or Weakness. Weight-Bearing Workouts Also Support Bone Health.

• Physical Activity Can Decrease Cancer-Related Fatigue, A Typical Adverse Effect Of Cancer Therapy. Engaging In Moderate Exercise Can Enhance Energy Levels And General Quality Of Life.

• Exercise Has A Beneficial Impact On Mental Health By Enhancing Mood And Decreasing Symptoms Of Anxiety

And Despair. This Is Particularly Important For Persons Facing The Emotional Difficulties Linked To A Cancer Diagnosis.

• Enhanced Immunological Function Is Linked To Exercise. Regular Physical Activity Can Be Beneficial For Those Receiving Cancer Therapies That May Compromise The Immune System.

• **Improved Respiratory Function:** For Persons With Lung Cancer, Engaging In Suitable Respiratory Exercises And Aerobic Activities Can Enhance Respiratory Function. This Is Crucial For Preserving Lung Capacity And General Respiratory Well-Being.

- **Pain Management:** Exercise Can Help In Alleviating Pain Related To Cancer And Its Therapies. It Can Decrease Muscular Tension, Enhance Joint Function, And Relieve Soreness.

- **Enhanced Treatment Tolerance:** Regular Physical Activity Has Been Associated With Increased Tolerance To Cancer Therapies. It Can Assist Individuals In Better Enduring The Adverse Effects Of Chemotherapy, Radiation Therapy, Or Surgery.

- Social Support And Engagement Can Be Fostered Through Group Fitness Activities Or Programs, Allowing For Social Connection And Support. This Communal Feeling Might Be Beneficial

For Persons Experiencing A Difficult Period.

Individuals With Lung Cancer Should Consult Their Healthcare Provider Before Initiating Any Fitness Regimen, Particularly While Undergoing Active Treatment. Exercise Should Be Customized Based On Individual Capabilities, Treatment Plans, And General Health Condition. Collaborating With Healthcare Professionals Such As Physical Therapists Or Exercise Specialists Can Help Create A Safe And Tailored Exercise Regimen For Persons With Lung Cancer.

Recipes and Meal Ideas

Of Course! Below Are Nutrient-Dense Recipes And Meal Suggestions That Can Be Customized To Accommodate The Preferences And Dietary Requirements Of Patients With Lung Cancer. These Are Broad Ideas. It Is Important To Take Into Account Individual Tolerances, Preferences, And Dietary Constraints. It Is Advisable To Seek Tailored Assistance From A Licensed Dietician Or Healthcare Expert.

Breakfast Ideas:

Berry and Yogurt Parfait:

• Layer Low-Fat Greek Yogurt With Mixed Berries (Blueberries,

Strawberries, Raspberries) And A Sprinkle Of Granola Or Chopped Nuts For Added Texture.

Oatmeal with Nut Butter and Banana:

• Cook Oats With Water Or Milk, And Top With A Dollop Of Almond Or Peanut Butter And Slices Of Banana. Add A Dash Of Cinnamon For Extra Flavor.

Lunch and Dinner Options:

Grilled Salmon With Quinoa And Roasted Vegetables:

• Grill Salmon And Serve It Over A Bed Of Cooked Quinoa. Roast A Variety Of Colorful Vegetables (Such As Broccoli,

Bell Peppers, And Carrots) For A Nutrient-Packed Side.

Chicken and Vegetable Stir-Fry:

• Stir-Fry Lean Chicken Breast With A Mix Of Colorful Vegetables (Snap Peas, Bell Peppers, Carrots, And Broccoli) In A Light Soy Or Teriyaki Sauce. Serve Over Brown Rice Or Quinoa.

Vegetarian Lentil Soup:

• Make A Hearty Lentil Soup With Lentils, Vegetables (Carrots, Celery, Tomatoes), And Flavorful Herbs And Spices. This Can Be A Nourishing And Easy-To-Digest Option.

Whole Grain Wrap With Turkey And Avocado:

• Create A Whole Grain Wrap With Lean Turkey Slices, Avocado, Lettuce, And Tomato. Add A Spread Of Hummus For Extra Flavor.

Snack Ideas:

Greek Yogurt with Fresh Fruit:

• Enjoy A Small Bowl Of Greek Yogurt With A Drizzle Of Honey And Fresh Fruit Slices (Such As Berries Or Kiwi).

Trail Mix With Nuts And Dried Fruit:

• Make A Homemade Trail Mix With A Mix Of Nuts (Almonds, Walnuts) And

Dried Fruit (Apricots, Raisins) For A Satisfying And Energy-Boosting Snack.

Dessert and Treats:

Baked Apples With Cinnamon:

• Core and Slice Apples, Sprinkle With Cinnamon, And Bake Until Tender. Top With A Dollop Of Greek Yogurt For A Healthy Dessert Option.

Dark Chocolate-Dipped Strawberries:

• Melt Dark Chocolate And Dip Fresh Strawberries For A Sweet Treat That Provides Antioxidants.

Ensure Meal Planning Includes A Diverse Range Of Foods, A Balanced Combination Of Nutrients, And

Controlled Portion Sizes. These Dishes Are Customizable According To Individual Dietary Choices And Limits. It Is Crucial To Stay Hydrated By Drinking Water Consistently Throughout The Day. Seek Guidance From Healthcare Specialists Or A Trained Dietician For Tailored Counsel According To Individual Requirements And Situations.

Conclusion

Ultimately, A Lung Cancer Diagnosis Presents Considerable Obstacles, Although Appropriate Nutrition, Physical Activity, And Supportive Treatment Are Crucial For Disease Management And Enhancing Quality Of Life.

An Adequately Balanced Diet With Fruits, Vegetables, Lean Proteins, Whole Grains, And Healthy Fats Can Enhance The Immune System, Improve Treatment Outcomes, And Alleviate Treatment-Induced Side Effects. It Is Crucial To Prioritize Maintaining A Healthy Weight, Remaining Well-Hydrated, And

According To Individual Dietary Requirements And Preferences.

Regular Physical Activity Is Crucial For Those Diagnosed With Lung Cancer. Physical Activity Can Enhance Physical Function, Cardiovascular Health, Muscle Strength, Mood, And General Well-Being. Customized Exercise Regimens Can Assist Individuals In Coping With Medication Adverse Effects, Minimizing Fatigue, And Improving Treatment Endurance.

During The Cancer Treatment Process, It Is Essential For Individuals To Collaborate Closely With Their Healthcare Team, Which May Include Oncologists, Registered Dietitians, Physical Therapists, And Other

Supportive Care Specialists. Collaboratively, They Can Create Customized Nutrition And Fitness Regimens Tailored To Individual Requirements To Enhance Overall Health Results.

Ultimately, When Faced With A Lung Cancer Diagnosis, Incorporating A Holistic Strategy With Adequate Nutrition, Consistent Physical Activity, And Thorough Supportive Measures Can Assist Individuals In Managing Their Experience With Increased Resilience, Vigor, And Health.

THE END